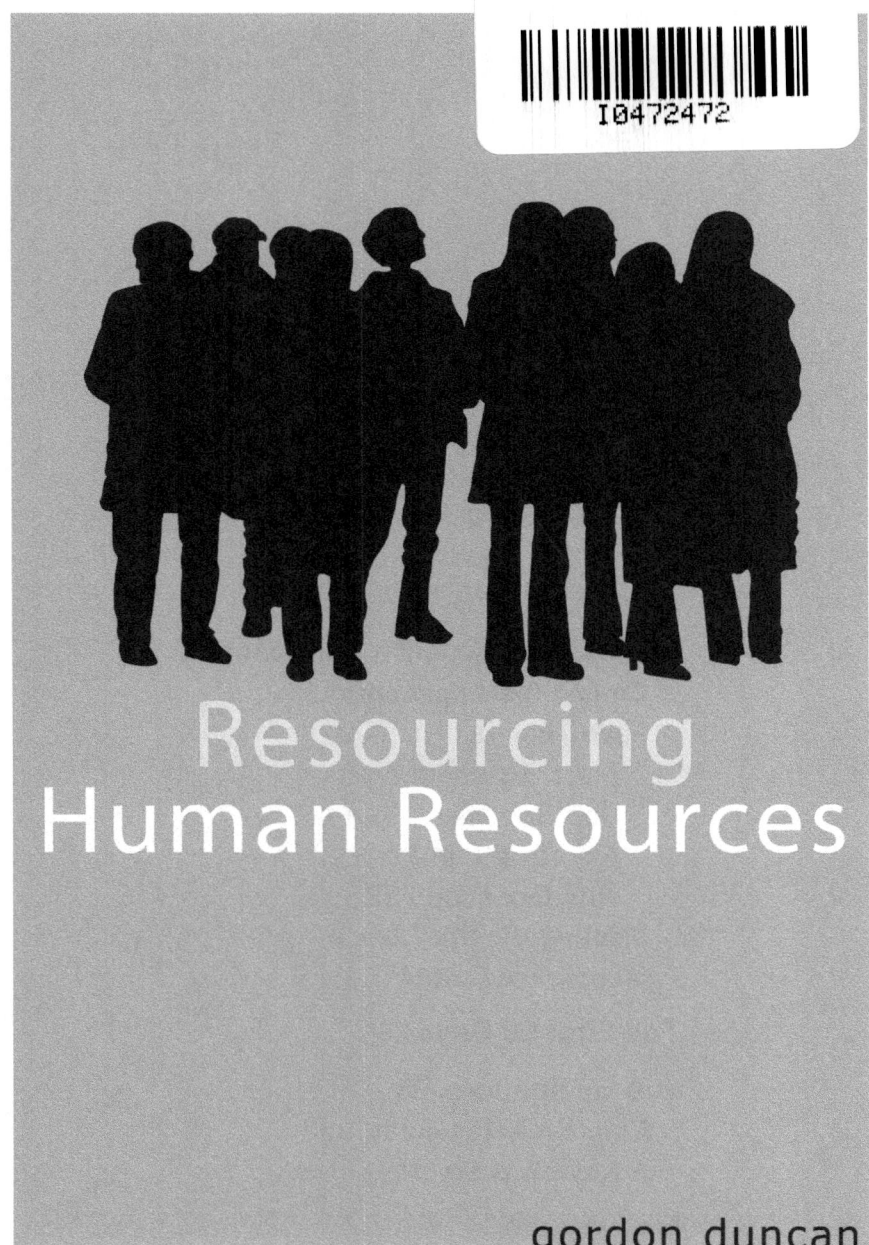

Resourcing
Human Resources

gordon duncan

Table of Contents

Introduction

In my twenty plus years in the education/sales/optometric/consulting worlds, I've noticed one fundamental challenge: staffing and retaining quality staff.

Even when I was a green school teacher a million years ago, I quickly realized that my principal had the daunting task of finding incredible teachers and convincing them to stay in the educational field. Most administrators continually have to overcome those obstacles despite their best efforts.

Understandably, many business owners either employ folks permanently (ala office manager) or hire folks specifically (ala consultant) to handle their hiring. Most folks just don't have time for it.

But if you either can't afford to spend the money or if you would rather just save a few bucks, this book is intended to help you. In it, you'll find ideas ranging from where to find quality applicants to how to conduct efficient interviews to how to retain quality employees.

We hope the book helps, and we hope you enjoy your business all the more because of it. Thanks for investing your valuable time into this book. We never take that for granted.

Gordon Duncan
Practice Progress
April, 2013

Finding Quality Applicants

It doesn't matter if you have the greatest job in the world that pays the greatest salary in the world if you cannot find the right applicants.

There is nothing more frustrating than spending an entire day interviewing a dozen people only to realize at closing time that you pretty much wasted the last few hours of your life and that you are no closer to hiring someone than you were when you began.

Those kinds of days happen when you have awful applicants in front of you. Those kinds of days are relieved when you find a quality pool to interview.

So how do you get a quality pool?

Well, we would like to offer several options for you, but first, let's start with a word of caution.

Word of Caution

For years, the standard way to get people to apply for a job was to pay for an ad in the local newspaper. Now days, at least you get an online ad to coincide with the print ad, but let's be honest.

Classified ads are expensive.

Let me give you an example. Take a mid-ranged metropolitan area like Raleigh, NC. Even if you only go with a one-day, Sunday ad (the highest circulation to get the highest impact), you are going to pay at least $299 for that ad.

So basically, for $300, you can place an ad and get folks to email, fax, or mail in resumes.

But who has an extra $300 these days?

Don't get me wrong; you can get quality applicants that way. Presumably, you get folks who are readers and folks who are looking diligently for a job.

But most of the time, it ain't worth $300.

So what is the best option? Free. Let's talk about finding quality applicants at no cost.

Finding Applicants for Free

Craigslist. If you have never been on it, get on it. If you have never placed an ad on it for a job opening, do it now. It is simple, and even better, it is free.

So first, let's talk about why it is your best option, and then we'll talk about how to do it.

Why Craigslist is Best

The reason Craigslist is your best resource for finding quality applicants is pretty simple. It is free to you and open to the world. Let me give you an example.

I was hired by a local eye doctor to help him fill a front desk position that had recently opened. His front desk gal gave the ubiquitous two-week notice, and he was in a rush to get the position filled.

He had hired me because he didn't want to give up a day of seeing patients in order to hire someone. But since hiring a consultant cost money, he wanted to save money going forward. Makes sense.

I suggested Craigslist as opposed to the usual newspaper ad in order to save money.

Now the next statement I'm going to make may seem like an exaggeration, and if you have never used Craigslist, you might think I'm lying, but I'm not.

Two hours after posting the job listing, I had over 100 resumes. In fact, I had to take down the ad just to go through those 100 to see if I had a quality pool. Fortunately, out of those 100, I had at least 10 people who I wanted to interview, and I had at least 3-4 applicants who had experience and seemed to fit the bill perfectly.

Now, as a qualifier, you might not get 100 resumes in the first hour, but you will probably get 100 within the first 48 hours.

And those 100 resumes won't cost you a dime.
With that in mind, let's find out how to post a job opening on Craigslist, let's

make sure you protect your identity, and let's make sure you know how to do it without costing you a dime.

Let's do it.

How to Do It

Some of you might be completely comfortable with Craigslist already. If you are, this section will be a refresher. If you want though, you can skip to the next chapter. If not, welcome to posting jobs on Craigslist.

Believe it or not, posting a job opening on Craigslist is pretty simple. Let's keep it obvious and simple.

Log on to www.craigslist.com.

What that will do is it will take you to a site where you can choose your state and the closest metropolitan area to you within that state. For the sake of example, let's choose Fredericksburg, VA. That would take you to here: http://fredericksburg.craigslist.org/.

On that page, you'll see over to the left a heading entitled, "post to classifieds". Click on it.

Once you are there, Craigslist will begin asking you a series of questions. The first of which is:

What type of posting is this?

Click "job offered", and then the page will ask you to agree to their guidelines. If you can, then click "I will abide by these guidelines" and move forward.

There you will choose out of a myriad of types of jobs. Pick the one that best describes your field. Again, for sake of example, let's click "admin/office jobs" to describe your position.

Here is where the real work happens. Let me make some very specific suggestions. This page will ask to give a "posting title" and a "specific location".

Make that title incredibly specific to weed out folks. If you are an eye care provider, then say, "Front Desk Position for Busy Eye Doctor Needed". I'm afraid that sounds like it was written for a 3rd grader, but here is the truth. It needs to be.

Keep it simple, and answer as many questions as you can in the title.

Once you get to an email address, you have two options. Either put in your real email or go to yahoo and make a fake one. Don't worry. Craigslist protects your email address if you click "anonymize", but I have known folks to create a "generic@yahoo.com" email address just to make sure.

The next step is to fill out the "Posting Description". Here, give as much information as you can about the position you are offering. Think through these things.

How much experience is required if any?

Mention whether this is a position that can grow into others.

Without speaking to specifics, offer some of the benefits that accompany the job like vacation, retirement, and sick days.

Speak to the office environment and office location - even mention local restaurants and other businesses nearby that might make the job convenient for applicants.

Then, fill out the compensation portion. I would suggest a range here. Give yourself some freedom and leeway without committing to a specific number.

Check the specifics below the compensation section, proofread, then proofread again, and if you are satisfied, click the continue button.

Now, you have an opportunity to add an image. Examples to consider would be your company logo, your office, and perhaps even the actual workspace that your new employee would occupy. Either way, postings with images get more and better applicants.

If you are pleased with your image, you can click the "publish" button. This, however, is not your last step. Clicking the "publish" button will trigger an activation email. If you don't check your email and click on the link, then your posting will not go live.

Once you complete the process, you job posting will available for folks to view, and the resumes will start coming in at a rapid pace.

But I would recommend one more step. Take that Craigslist link, and share it across your other pages. Include it on your webpage, your company's Facebook page, and even on sites like Pinterest.

Believe it or not, within the next 24-48 hours, you will receive a ton of resumes. In one example, I received over 100 resumes in the first 4 hours of posting the ad. I posted it on a Monday morning and was overwhelmed with applicants by noon.

I would suggest once you get a large enough pool of applicants to take the ad down. Otherwise, your email will be blowing up all day long. Don't worry, you can repost the ad again if you need to, so you won't have to duplicate the work. Seriously, you will not believe how many emails you will get in a short amount of time. Folks need jobs, and what they really need is good jobs which you are offering.

Once the resumes come in, the question will be, "What to do next?" Let's answer that question.

What to Do Next?

I'm old school. Once I have my pool of resumes, I print them out, but do it however you want. The next step is to weed down the applicants. Here is my suggestion.

Make your first pass through your resumes quick. Put a couple of things in mind that will help you create two stacks of resumes. Name one stack "Nope" and the other stack "Maybe".

How do you decide which is which? Well, I usually have two criteria: proximity and experience. If folks have specific or even cross-similar experience, they are a keeper. What I mean by cross-similar experience is whether or not folks have done anything that might enable them to do your job well. If they live 100 miles away, they aren't.

Once, I managed a large medical office. I was out doing some shopping, and the gal at the checkout counter was excellent at her job. I saw her be gracious to a troublesome customer. She answered a question from another employee. She gave me full attention and even asked a few questions as I checked out. Her place of work was not a medical clinic, but she modeled every characteristic I would want in a front desk employee. So as I checked, I gave her my card and told her that if she wanted to apply for a job to call me the next day.

She anchored my front desk for the next several years. As you go through these resumes, actual experience in your field is valuable, but every now and then, you want to grab someone with similar experience and give them a chance. Typically, these valuable employees can even be hired for a bit less than a job-specific experienced employee, and you do just as well.

So you now have your two stacks. The "nopes" you are done with and the "maybes" deserve your attention. Now what? I usually try to get the stack down to 10-12 folks because that is the number I can interview in a day. You may not have a whole day to give to the process, so whether or not you are extending the process over several days or one, give yourself a nice pool to choose from.

Still, how do you get to the 10-12? Here are several things to consider.

Industry-specific experience has got to be prioritized. If they have done your job before, you have got to spend time on that resume. If you have those, ask these questions.

Why are the leaving their current job?

Have they hopped around from job to job too much?

Have they worked for folks that you can contact to get more info?

If they have cross-similar experience, ask the same questions to yourself above, but also ask a few more.

Will this job ask them to change work habits, approach, and maybe even work dress?

Will this job put too much of a stress on them in light of other things in their resume?

What would motivate them to leave their present field to join yours?

Once you have your 10-12 candidates set, keep a Group B set of folks ready in case you have to do this again. But now that you have your 10-12, let's move to the actual interviews.

Interviewing Quality Applicants

Hopefully, this process has given you a fantastic pool of applicants. Whether you got them from Craigslist, the paper, or some other avenue, now comes the hard part: interviewing. Let's take it step by step.

Calling the Applicants

Yes, call them. Someone needs to speak to your applicants before they take up your valuable time. Now you might wonder, "Well, if I call them, I have to bring them in, so why do I have to call them?" Let me explain.

Once you have that list of 10-12 candidates, call each of them. Don't bring in anyone you haven't spoken with on the phone. Approach them this way.

Call and ask for them by name. If they don't answer, leave a detailed message and ask them to get back in touch with you that day. Unless they are out and out rock stars, don't save a spot for them (or maybe save a spot but only until the end of the day). Availability equals possibility.

Again, in the message, do not tell them that you want them to come in for an interview. Just tell them that you would like to follow up with them about the resume they submitted for the ad.

Whenever you get them, whether immediately or on a call back, listen for a few things. Tell them that you would like to ask them a few follow up questions. Now, these questions can have a point, but more than anything, you are making a quick assessment of the person's phone skills.

Typical questions to ask might be:

'So, tell me about..." and then ask about the specific job experience referenced on their resume.

Ask them what attracted them to this job.

Ask them what would distinguish them from the other candidates.

These questions are important, and more than likely, you will repeat them face to face. But before you actually invite them in for an interview, you have got to pay attention to a few things.

Do they speak in a way that you feel will represent your company/office is well?

Are they able to articulate their answers clearly and in an efficient manner?

Do they have a trustworthy demeanor in their voice? If they don't have those things, then you have to decide whether it is worth your time to bring them into an interview.

The phone will teach you a lot and will weed out a ton of candidates. But nothing can replace interviewing them face to face.

Face Time

Interviews face to face cannot be replaced. Typically, when I line up a day of interviews, I schedule them about thirty minutes apart. But once they arrive, I let them wait. I want my staff to observe how they handle the down time.

Do they read?
Do they fidget?
Do they pick their nose?

I don't know what they do, but my staff knows to watch. If I can get an extra moment to observe them before they notice me, I do the same thing. I watch.

Before bringing them into your interview space, set up a few things.

First, make sure your interview room is either visible or has a door open. You do not want to interview someone behind a closed door. It is a lawsuit waiting to happen.

I always let them enter the room first, and I always interview folks at a table with four chairs. I love just watching how people either decide which chair they want or ask which chair they should take.

But face to face is the time to ask the questions to help you determine who to hire, and that is a non-negotiable. Many of the same points and questions apply now as they did on the phone, but in this arena, you get real-time feedback as to the competency and potential of this employee.

These don't have to follow any specific order, but here are a few categories of questions to consider (including actual questions to throw at your candidate).

Past Experience

Again, all the information about where your applicants have worked is on their resume, but more important than where they have worked is how they speak about where they have worked. Look for respect and honesty related to their past jobs. Ask them:

Tell me about Such-and-Such job. What did you like about that job?

What did that job opportunity teach you that might prepare you for this job?

Why did you leave that job?

Why are you looking for a new job?

Tell me about a situation where you learned from a mistake you made on the job. Were you able to either correct it or prevent it from happening again? If so, how?

How do you think your past experience qualifies you or enables you to do this job?

Which of these jobs do you think you would be available for rehire if you reapplied?

Which of these jobs would you feel comfortable with our contacting for reference?

Bottom line: Encourage your applicants to speak specifically about their past employments. More than likely, who you are hiring is not going to work with you until the day you die, so their interaction with you about past jobs is going to give you an indication of what their attitude towards your office/business will be like.

One final note: I have seen business owners become overwhelmed with applicants with great relatable experience. And in the process, they don't ask thorough enough questions. Don't be blinded by a good resume. Vet often. Vet always.

Job Specifics

In this next portion of the interview, you want to explain the job you are offering in as detailed a manner as possible. That requires some preparation on your part.

But before we get there, let me offer this one note. After speaking to the candidate about their past experience, you may have already decided that you don't want to hire them.

Don't waste your time, then. Ask them if they have any questions about the job they are applying for, answer them, and then thank them for applying. Move on if you know you are not going to hire someone.

Having said that, how much have you thought about the job that you are offering? It may be a job that has been in your office/practice for years so you haven't thought much about it lately or it may be a brand new position. My advice: Think about it this way.

Have you ever hired an employee that you thought was just going to be perfect

for a position, but once they started,
they were a fish out of water?
Sometimes that happens because they
made themselves out to be something
they weren't in the interview, but
sometimes that happens because the
position was inaccurately presented and
detailed in the interview. Ask yourself:

Is my presentation of this position
accurate and comprehensive enough to
match the perfect person to this job?

Does my presentation of this position
need adjusting in light of recent changes
in staffing, technology, location, etc.?

Does my presentation of this position
eliminate any surprises that might await
the person who fills it?

Are there common factors for why
people have left this position that I have
neglected to address or to mention?

As you walk through the position, be
sure to give the interviewer an
opportunity to ask questions.

To be honest, I am completely
unimpressed with anyone who doesn't

have follow up questions. In fact, there are some parts of the job that I explain vaguely in order to give the applicant an opportunity to ask questions. If they don't see those areas, then they are telling you something about themselves.

Personal Life

When it comes down to it, you want to know this question: Can this PERSON do this job?

Tons of folks can apply and interview well, but whether or not a particular person can do a job is only discovered as they walk through the door. So what can you do before hand to better know the individual in front of you?

Legally, you cannot ask a bunch of personal questions. In fact, you almost can't ask anything about their family, children, and home life. So, you have got to be creative. Here are a few questions/starters to get you there.

"Hey, I like to get to know you a little, tell me about yourself."

This question lets you know how free this person is with talking about themselves. They may open right up, and if they do, you quickly learn who they are and what they are like. If they say everything but something personal, you have two deductions to make: They are either extremely private or their homelife might be one that they don't want you to know much about. Neither is bad, but either way, you are learning.

The opener is pretty common, so it is key you ask questions that folks aren't use to answering. Next, try this one on for size.

"If you had a weekend to yourself, what would you do?"

I love that question. It takes folks by surprise a bit. Most folks don't have weekends to themselves because of life commitments. So having a weekend free means that whatever it is that folks are busy with has been removed. Folks have a tendency to mention that with the question. Along the way, you also find out a little bit about their interests which is always revealing towards a person's personality.

I've had folks answer that question in a variety of ways.

"Oh, with my three kids, I never get a weekend free."

"Well, if my sorry ex-husband would come pick the kids up like he is supposed to, then I could have a free weekend."

"I would go running."

"I would go to the movies."

"I usually hang out with buddies."

All of these offer you a ton of options for follow up. But let's say they are still tight-lipped about themselves. Again, they are not under any legal obligation to say anything personal, but you want to know who you are going to hire. This next question is simple, but it reveals a lot.

"Do you read a lot? If so, tell me about the last few books you've read."

Spiritual books let you know you are hiring someone religious.

Political books let you know you are hiring someone political.

And on and on. Sometimes, folks will say, "Goodness, I never have time to read." Then you ask, "Why not?" But no matter the answer, you learn a lot by asking about reading habits.

The one question I love though is this one:

"So tell me, all things being equal, why should I hire you above the other 100 applicants I have."

Most folks can't answer it. Someone will say, "I really need a job." Some will say, "Because I have the best experience." And some will not know what to say.

One time, I had an applicant start the interview by saying, "Well, you can stop looking right now. I'm the best candidate for the job. No need to look any further."

I must admit I was intrigued by their confidence and hoped they could back it up. So I said, "Awesome. Tell me why."

Sadly, they couldn't answer. Honestly, they stumbled around for the next 5 minutes, and we moved on with a very brief interview.

So, no matter what you ask, be wise in pursuing personal questions, but figure out how to ask them without getting in trouble. The ones here are pretty innocuous. Use them if they help, but if you don't, you have to figure out some way to get to know the people you are considering hiring.

Any Questions

Yeah, I know. Everyone asks at the end of the interview, "So, do you have any questions for me?" This is standard, bringing the interview to a close type question. But let me offer this: Don't skip this. Make a big deal out of it. Here is why.

You want to hire someone who engages with what you say, can process in real time, and take thoughts through logical progressions.

When an applicant says, "No, you just about covered it all," I am not impressed. Why? Because they are not trying hard enough to make an impression. Don't get me wrong, I've hired people who had nothing to ask, but an applicant who can put together a thoughtful question to either extend the conversation or pursue next steps is always someone worth considering heavily.

Meeting the Staff

Please do not hire anyone who you
haven't introduced to your staff. You
may have already made up your mind,
but if they don't fit with your staff, they
are going to be poison.

Typically, when I'm doing the carwash of
interviews, I take the applicants who
have potential to meet the staff. Either, I
walk through them through the office
and personally introduce them, or I ask
the applicant to wait where I'm
interviewing and then bring in the staff
one by one to talk to them.

I let the staff know at the beginning of
the day that I might do this. I ask them
to get to know the applicants as well as
they can in those few minutes. This
serves several purposes.

One, bringing the staff in on the process
lets the staff know that you find their
opinion and input valuable.

Two, bringing the staff in on the process
lets you make a very informed decision
before you say, "You're hired."

Three, bringing the staff in on the process also gives you a better chance of getting to know the applicant personally. This one is crucial, and let me tell you why.

Typically, when staff and applicants talk, they have personal conversations that you could never have. Just casually, they are sharing things about themselves and asking questions. If you process with your staff afterwards, you will know so much more about your candidate.

I've had staff say both sides of the decision after meeting someone. They've said, "She is the one," and they have said, "Nope. No way." It is still your call, but bringing your staff in enables you to make your most informed decision.

Making the Call

Make the call. You might ask, "Well, what do I do if my staff wants one person and I want the other?" If that is the case, ask yourself a few questions.

Is my favorite so much better than the staff's that going against their choice is worth it? If your choice is clearly heads and shoulders above the other, then hire that person and explain to the staff how much you appreciate their input and give them a sense of the intangibles in which they might not have been aware.

Just prepare yourself for an extra staffing challenge. Your choice might be or might become a hall of famer; that's fine. Just walk the staff through it. But you'll find that if you have a competent staff, they often pick the right person.

I remember once sorting through 100 resumes, conducting 12 interviews, and bring back 3 candidates for a second interview. I had tiered the candidates in my mind as 1,2,3, but I wanted the staff to give their input.

My number 1 was completely shot down. No one gave a real reason other than, "Something just didn't feel right." I was completely suspicious of the staff, and began to doubt both their ability and their integrity.

My number 2 was their number 1, and they begged me to hire her.

My number 3 was their close second, and all of them said that if things didn't work out with their top choice, they felt confident that this applicant would work.

So, I had a decision to make. The staff unanimously loved number 2, and felt as strong about their distaste for my number 1. Choosing against them was going to be an uphill climb. Number 2 was not that far off though.

So I called 1 and 3 and told them that we liked them both but decided to go with someone else. I called number 2, and she quickly accepted the job.

Well, believe it or not, number 2 lasted 2 days and had to quit because she couldn't acquire adequate kid coverage. Number 3 took the job and took off.

I say all that to say that the staff felt intricately a part of the process, and it helped. When their choice didn't work out, they apologized. When the next person came in, they worked twice as hard to get her assimilated. In the end, the staff became united and worked well together. Going forward, old and new worked well together by all of them taking part in the process.

The First 90 Days

Now, I have read the books that speak against 90 day evaluations, and I'll be honest. I agree with many of them. But I will also say this.

In the world of hourly employees, you do not have any choice but to start each new employee off on a 90 day evaluation.

Let me explain. A 90 day evaluation works like this. Any new hire must work 90 calendar days before they can enjoy the benefits of a full-time employee.

Hire these employees, and let them know this. Let them know that the next 90 days are an evaluation period. You will provide every measure of training that you can and that the staff will do the same. Tell them that your office door is always open, and that you will want them to succeed.

If all goes well, you will sit down with them in 90 days and give them a full evaluation. You will walk through their strengths and weaknesses and offer them a full-time job, and hopefully they are going to accept.

No employee should work 90 days and then find out that they don't have a job.

Let them know that at any time in the 90 days, either of you can walk away clean. Those are the terms of the 90 day hire. At any point during that time, you can walk up and say, "This is not working out. Thanks." And likewise, without any notice, they can do the same. In the first 90 days, they are an interim hire.

Day 91, they are a full-time employee. They can have insurance, retirement, and any other benefit you offer. If you provide vacation and sick days based on days worked, their 90 days goes towards that, and they will continue to accrue them going forward.

But these 90 days are essential. Anyone who will not accept these terms is not someone you need to hire. Not in this environment. You can have 100 resumes in your hand in 24 hours.

If you are still skeptical, just consider the cost of adding an employee to insurance or a retirement account. Add in your time and your money in the process. If you have to then call all of those folks and cancel or change coverage because your new hire quit after the first week, you are burning time and money.

And besides, any employee that won't work hard to earn their job in 90 days is not someone you want anyway. And an employee who works 90 days and earn those benefits will appreciate them more.

Job Evaluations

I mentioned a 90 day evaluation above, and these are the same as your yearly evaluations. We spoke of this briefly in the original "Practice Progress" book, but the importance is worth reviewing.

Evaluations are absolutely necessary. There must be a yearly anticipated time where staff sit down with you and evaluate themselves and are evaluated. And that is the key: employees must evaluate themselves before you sit down with them.

I suggest giving them an evaluation form. There is one below or you can make up another. Give them some number evaluation system (1-5, 1-10), and then tell them to evaluate themselves and give an explanation for why they gave themselves that number.

They then bring that form with them to the evaluation where you have filled out a form for them from your perspective. Then walk through each step or characteristic with them. Ask them what they gave themselves and why, and then counter with your own evaluation. When there is a great difference, there is usually a great conversation.

By the end of your time together, you should have the staff person sign and date two copies of your evaluation: one to keep and one for their employee file.

But let your staff know this one thing: evaluations are not attached to raises. They can be, but they aren't automatic. There is nothing worse than a staff person who thinks they should get a raise every year. So tell them, "Gang, sometimes raises are handed out at evaluations, but they shouldn't be expected each year. Raises are based on two things: improvement and financial availability. If you improve this year and we have the financial resources, we'll give you a raise. If we don't have both of those, we can't do raises. You might get a raise mid-year or even mid-month if improvement and availability are there. Please understand though: evaluations are not the guaranteed raise season."

Tell folks this when you are hiring them. Remind them throughout the year, and inform them one more time before you start the evaluation process.

To help or give a guideline, attached a sample evaluation.

Employee Review

Rank Yourself in the
Following categories from 1-5
1 is the lowest and 5 is the highest
With each category, include an explanation

EMPLOYEE NAME:
SIGNATURE:

1. Punctuality: _____

    Explain:

2. Appearance: _____

    Explain:

3. Job Knowledge: _____

    Explain:

4. Efficiency: _____

    Explain:

5. Accuracy: _____

    Explain:

6. Dependability: _____

    Explain:

7. Innovativeness: _____

    Explain:

8. Professionalism: _____

    Explain:

9. Patient Interaction: _____

    Explain:

10. Leadership: _____

    Explain:

11. Staff Relations: _____

    Explain:

A Review Story

Establishing reviews if you haven't done them will sometimes cause some bumps, but it will also help turn some employees around. That was exactly what happened in one office.

After a dozen or so years, the owner decided it was time to give the staff a review. She wanted them to have a sense of where they were, and she wanted them to begin working towards goals, so she brought me in to work with her staff.

Things did not get off to a good start. As soon as I walked in, the staff began to murmur, and the most senior employee made no bones about it. She told me that I wasn't needed.

Being used to such welcoming, I continued on, gathered the staff, and explained the process. Just like above, I handed out the review, asked them to assign themselves a number, and explained their evaluation. The owner and I told them that we would also be reviewing them and that we would be meeting with each staff person individually to compare notes and sketch out a plan going forward.

And, believe it or not, the staff was quite receptive. They were honest evaluators of their skills and weaknesses. They came in pretty hesitant, but they left encouraged and renewed to do their job well.

Until the most senior employee walked in the door...

She came in defensive and defiant. I calmly explained to her that the owner and I wanted to hear her evaluation and explanation, and then we would respond with ours. Following those two things, we would outline a plan for her growth in the company.

She responded by handing us her written evaluation. In each category, she gave herself a 5 out of 5 and offered no explanation. She must have spent less than 30 seconds on the entire process.

I asked her to give an explanation as to why she put so little time into the evaluation, and she said she was good at what she did and didn't have any areas of improvement. She had worked at that office so long that she could run it by herself and didn't need any input from me as to how to improve.

The owner and I were faced with a dilemma: an obstinate employee who didn't want to participate in our process.

So I took the reins. This is what I told her. "Well, since you already do every aspect of this job perfectly, and there is no room for improvement, we are going to let you go."

She awoke from her confident slumber very quickly. "Let me go? Why?"

I responded, "I think we are holding you back. If you can run this office without any help, and you have no room to improve, and you don't need to participate in our process, we want to free you up to go find a bigger and better job."

She broke down crying and asked for an opportunity to re-evaluate herself and come back. She did just that, and the owner gained a better employee.

Now, we both know things don't always work out that well. You may very well have to let some folks go or work incredibly hard with a difficult employee to get them there, but you won't even begin to be able to start that process unless you are giving regularly scheduled evaluations.

Motivations

As we wrap up, there is a reality, no matter what kind of business you own. Your staff needs constant and continual motivation. You would like to think that a regular paycheck would be motivation enough, but it isn't.

Creatively, you need to come up with some type of bonus, spiff, or motivation system above a paycheck.

Now, I know your rebuttal. Some of you try to keep payroll at a certain % (typically 20-25%) of your overall expenses. I highly recommend this. But some of you might think, "If I pay out a bunch of bonuses, I can't keep to this goal."

This is true unless your bonuses are based on improved revenue. No matter what you spiff your staff on, make their bonuses based on your having more money in the bank.

If you deposit more, and then spiff them a small % of that improvement, then you will actually see your payroll %'s drop.

Your staff will find motivation. You will have more money in the bank. And everyone will be all the more happy because of a bonus system.

Now, no book can cover a bonus system for every type of office, so in conclusion, your find several appendices covering everything from general business to specific types of offices. Some of these were mentioned in the original "Practice Progress" book, and a few are new and adapted. Either way, we hope they help, and we hope you find greater enjoyment in your business.

Appendix I - Deposit Bonus

This is an all staff bonus that directly helps you put money in your pocket while motivating your staff. Here is how it works.

- Create a 12 month chart from the prior year that lists what your deposits were for each month
- Then project 5, 10, 15, and 20% growth.
- Affix a value for each employee if they meet this goal.

Before I show you an example, let me address a few fears. You may not want your employees to know your deposits, but I will say they already do. They have a sense of how money your office takes in, and it is probably an overly-skewed sense. Go ahead and tell them the truth. For most of them, it will be a reality check.

Secondly, don't worry about paying out these bonuses. You only have to pay them out when your office improves its deposits from last year and the payout

for most offices is only a tiny % of the
extra money you have put in the bank.
Let me demonstrate for you.

Deposit Goals – 20xx

Last Yr. Dep ($150)	5% ($100) 20% ($175)	10% ($125)	15%
Jan	66,327 79,592	69,643	72,960	76,276
Feb	71,754 86,105	75,342	78,929	82,517
Mar	80,858 97,030	84,901	88,944	92,987
April	87,763 105,316	92,151	96,539	101,042
May	77,089 92,507	80,943	84,798	88,652
June	80,223 96,268	84,234	88,256	92,256
July	71,673 86,008	75,257	78,840	82,424
Aug	75,674 90,809	79,458	83,241	87,025
Sep	76,026 91,231	79,827	83,629	87,430
Oct	81,950 98,340	86,048	90,145	94,143
Nov	62,457 74,948	65,580	68,703	71,826
Dec	67,525 81,030	70,901	74,278	77,654

Okay, let's take this in. In January of last year, you deposited $66,327 with a staff of 5 people. With a 5% increase of deposits to $69,643, you will give each one of those staff $100. Do the math.

- You deposited $3,316 more in that month than you did in the same time period last year.
- You paid out $500 in bonuses.
- The net for you is $2,816.

Let's say that in that same month you have killer growth and increase your deposits by 20%. Do the math.

- You deposited $13,265 more in that month than you did in the same time period last year.
- You paid out $875 in bonuses.
- The net for you is $12,390.

This is a win/win for you. When your month is chugging along, and you know that if your staff works just a little bit harder filling the schedule or they need a little motivation to sell frames or contacts, this is how you get them to where they need to be.

This is also where your projections come into place. If your staff is aware of these numbers and they know how to project, they motivate themselves. But your input and your awareness of the numbers always helps as well.

For example, if it is day 15 out of 20 in the month, and the staff see that they are falling a bit short of receiving their 5% bonus, then they know that with a little extra effort, they can hit their numbers. I mean, what else is going to motivate them? If you have two business days left to go, or even just one, what is going to motivate your staff to pack their Friday schedule? Nothing really. In fact, without something like this in place, you'll notice your Friday schedules becoming more and more light. Your encouragement to them with a desire to pay them their bonus helps them work harder.

I have seen this exact scenario take place. One time, I was at an office on a Friday morning. I knew that there were several openings in the afternoon. Two patients called in a row asking about available exams, and the response they received was that there were openings next week. I thought, "What about today?"

Well, without some motivation to hit a number like a deposit, I'm afraid people are going to default to what is easiest. But if the staff is working towards getting $100, those two phone calls will be a blessing (and worth somewhere around $600). If you don't see this motivating your staff, you probably need new staff.

Appendix II – Bonus Systems for Eye Care Professionals

Photo Bonus

Not every office has a camera taking routine photos, but they have become the standard of care. Some offices just build those photos into their exam which is fine, but you are not being reimbursed for those by most insurance companies. So many practices offer a routine photo for diagnostic purposes at an extra cost of anywhere from $25 to $50.

Spending money above and beyond a copay is understandably not an easy thing to convince a patient to do. But the photo gives you as a doctor real, helpful information about your patient's ocular health. Motivating your workup person to ask your patients for this additional service is not an easy thing to do. So spiff them to motivate them.

Look at your averages over the last year, create a chart much like the deposit chart with projected % improvements, and spiff them. Very little else will get your tech to go above and beyond their normal patterns and areas of comfortability. Imagine spiffing your tech $50 after they sell 25 more photos than last month at $25 a pop. The math is easy. You deposited $1,250, spiffed $50, netted $1,200, and your patients received more comprehensive eye care.

One last note on camera spiffs. It might help your techs if you give them a script to memorize and adapt at first. They just flat out may need the help. Here is one that you can adapt as needed.

"Retinal photographs are the standard of care chosen by Drs. _____ and _____ because they serve as a baseline for your ocular health. The Drs. recommend that all first time patients get them. Additional photos are only necessary when the Drs. feel that there is an issue to monitor. Despite the value of these photos, your insurance does not cover their cost, so there is an additional charge of $25. Can we take those photos for you today?"

Of course, your tech can customize this script once they grow comfortable with it, but getting them started with something like this is typically a big help.

Optical Bonus

The first and most important optical bonus you can implement is when your sellers move a number of frames consistent with your goals. For example, if you want to turn your frame board over 2.5 times a year, then figure out the number of frames that have to be sold in a year. Divide that by the weeks you are open and even go so far as to break down by day.

Understandably, your office more than likely closes for Thanksgiving and Christmas and Easter, so just go ahead and set your weeks of operation at 50. Let's use an office with 400 frames on the frame board for our example.

600 frames x 2.5 = 1,500 projected frames sold a year
1,500 frames divided by 50 weeks = 30 frames sold a week.
30 frames a week divided by 5 business days = 6 frames a day.

Now before we talk about spiffing these numbers, your first reaction might be, "What? I better sell more than 6 frames a day." First of all this is just a hypothetical, and secondly, and I hate to do this to you, check and see how many frames you sold last year.
Add up the total, divide by 250, and you'll probably be shocked. I hope not, but chances are you might be.

Either way, let's use these numbers for our examples: 30 frames a week and 6 a day. First of all, if your optical hits 30 a week, bonus them. Figure out the best number, but let's say you give your sellers $50 each week they hit their number. Don't panic; you are paying out $100 in bonuses (to two staff) only and if they sell 30 frames. The average frame price is probably $179 or so. Do the math. They sell $5,370 worth of frames and you pay out $100. It will be okay. The important thing is you want your sellers motivated.

I used to spiff my optical daily. Seriously. I would even let the benefits spread to the whole office. It worked like this. If the staff hit their daily numbers, I would buy the office breakfast. Or I would tier it; sell 2 more frames than your daily total, and everyone gets muffins!

Before you think that I went broke buying muffins, stop worrying. It always paid out. The staff had a couple of cheap options for breakfast. Typically it was donuts or muffins. So let's say my optical sold 8 frames one day. Average frame price was $179 so we sold $1,432 worth of frames. I would then spend $12 on muffins for the whole staff. Everyone was motivated, and everyone was fed. The steady (and increased sales) always made the cost of food worth it.

I have seen my staff absolutely kill themselves and then celebrate to get that last frame sale at the end of the day just so they could get muffins. I loved it. I encouraged it. Every day, I would walk in the office, verify the deposit, check to see if they hit their numbers, and then head out on my errands. I would make the deposit, and then I would pick up donuts for everyone. Life was good on those days.

Weekly Bonus

Weekly bonuses work the same way, of course. You need to sell your 30 frames per week, and you need to find a way to spiff your staff. Again, I encourage an all office spiff. Pick 4-5 affordable restaurants around you and make lunch the spiff. A great way to start a Monday is eating the lunch earned on Friday. And again, the cost is no big deal. Pizza, subs, etc are going to run you $50 or so for lunch. Your staff sold $5,370 worth of frames (30 x $179 avg frame price). In the long run, if your staff is consistently turning over their frame boards, $50 worth of pizza is no big deal.

An added bonus is that sharing the spiff with the whole staff will improve inter-office relations. No matter how hard you have worked to protect salary anonymity, your staff assumes the frame sellers make more money. I've seen this turn really ugly before. The front desk person who gets to eat subs because the frame sellers did their job well has one less thing to complain about.

Year's Supply of Contact Lens

At all times, you should know the % of your patients that are contact lens wearers. The easy way to do that is to walk through each month of last year and divide the number of contact lens evaluations by the total number of comprehensive eye exams. Most docs run somewhere between 25% - 33%, but I do know a few that are a bit higher.

Once you know that number, you should be able to set realistic expectations for how many years' supplies of contacts you want to sell each month. Put that in front of your front desk and techs, and spiff them if they hit that number. An organized, motivated mindset to sell a year's supply will definitively increase sells. I saw this demonstrated back in the gravy days. Let me explain.

Many years ago, back when sales reps could directly spiff docs for selling their products, we had a contact lens rep cut a deal with us. If we sold 200 year's supply of their brand of contacts in a 3 month period, the rep would take the entire staff to Ruth Chris steakhouse. In essence, the rep was offering to pay for

18 people to eat whatever they wanted at an incredibly high end restaurant if we pushed her contacts. Now of course, these types of practices are illegal these days, but guess what happened back then? We sold 200 year's supplies of her contact in 8 weeks…and the steak was very good; thank you very much. All it took was some motivation.

Now this is a good time to talk about retaining contact lens sells, so let me speak to that for a second. This issue is much like the issue in facing the big box stores. You cannot compete with 1-800-get your contacts cheap or the big box stores. Now, you can negotiate contact lens prices, and you should let your contact lens rep know that for the most part, they are all the same. You don't tell your patients that, but the differences aren't more than minimal.

Bottom line: if your rep doesn't negotiate, tell them you are finding a new lens or a new rep.

But back to retaining your contacts lens sells. You, your front desk, and your techs have got to be on the same page when it comes to selling contacts. You are always going to offer your patients your best deal by selling year's supplies.

Now, I know in this economy, dropping $180 - $250 dollars at a time for contacts is a tough pill to swallow. But you have got to explain to your patients that this is their best deal. They will either nickel and dime it online and pay exorbitant shipping and handling or they can find a healthy price with you. Negotiate with your vendors. Some of them will ship directly to the patients with no cost. And you know what? 1-800-whatever is not going to replace a bad contact if you get one. You will. Your folks have got to make this effort.

Now, I know some docs who tell me that their patients buy all their contacts from them anyway, they just don't buy a year's supply at one time. Their patients call in 3-4 times a year, so there is no need to push it. If that is your situation, good for you, but there is one problem with that scenario. You are losing money. Let me explain.

Let's say your patient gets contacts from you 4 times a year: at their yearly exam, and every 3 months after that. Well, those 3 times that they call in throughout the year cost you money. Your employee answers the phone 3 times, pulls their chart/looks them up on the computer 3 times, orders their contacts 3 times, processes their orders when they come in 3 times, calls your patient back 3 times, and dispenses those contacts 3 times. Yeah, you received your patient's money for a year supply, but you wound up making a lot less money.

Maybe each of those interactions took 3 minutes of your employee's time. That employee makes $10 an hour. 3 minutes is worth $.50. Since your patient keeps calling in, you paid your employee $3.00 to process all of those orders which made your already thin profit on contacts even smaller.

Bottom Line: Teach your staff to sell year's supplies.

Appendix III – Bonus for Offices who File Insurance

Insurance Bonus

Most doctors do not manage their insurance person because they just don't know the inner workings of insurance. Additionally, I've known OD's who have kept horrible insurance people around because they just assumed that they couldn't find another and they feared what would happen income-wise if they didn't have someone in that spot for 2 weeks. Don't do that. ***Fire bad employees.***

Losing two weeks of insurance income is probably less than what you are losing by employing an insurance person who is not getting it done.

The good thing about an insurance bonus is that it is a built in accountability module. If they don't hit the numbers, they don't get a bonus, and you have questions to ask. And hear me on this: you must meet face to face with your insurance person each month. So much so, that you are familiar with your insurance balances in each age category (0-30, 31-60, etc). You need to be able to ask about specific outstanding balances.

For example, sometimes getting paid for post-op cataract work is incredibly hard. You might be owed over $400 for a single patient that is over 60 days old. You have got to know this and manage this, and I'll tell you why. I do not mean to impugn your insurance person, but there will always be a temptation to just write off difficult claims so as not to have too high of old balances. And in the big picture, if you are not managing these things, you will never know it. $400 in your write off total will probably not even be noticed. So here is how you spiff/manage your insurance person.

I suggest giving your insurance person $100 - $150 if all of their insurance totals 90 days and under are 97% or higher of their overall outstanding insurance. I know that sounds convoluted, so let me explain.

With this plan, only 3% of your entire outstanding insurance total is 91 days or older. 90 days is plenty of time for a claim to filed, fixed, and re-filed. A good insurance person can even get 3 filings in in 90 days. Any claim over 90 days is definitively in jeopardy of being collected, and your person has got to know what the issue is by that time. The formula for determining these numbers is as follows:

Current + (31–60) + (61-90) divided by insurance **total**

For example, let's say these are your outstanding insurance numbers.

(Current) $28,758.03 + **(31-60)** $1973.77 + **(61-90)** $366.79 = $31,098.59

Your Total Outstanding Insurance = $32,484.59

(All Insurance 90 days and Younger) $31,098.59 divided by **(Your Total Outstanding Insurance)** $32,484.59 = .957 or 96%

In this scenario, your insurance person would not receive a bonus for the month. The best idea is to get your numbers presently, plug them in, and find out the health of your outstanding Insurance A/R. As soon as you do this, you are probably going to realize that implementing a plan like this is going to require a massive cleanup of your outstanding insurance.

Sit down with your insurance person and speak about every single over 90 claim and any 61-90 day claim (as they will be over 90 very soon). You might be surprised to find out that you have claims on the books that are years old. More than likely, you aren't ever going to collect them, and you will just have to write them off. Claims that are a year old, or are otherwise seen as uncollectable, just have to go off the books.

Clean the numbers up, and start your insurance person off with some of hitting their goal. But your insurance person can only write off the claims that you approve. They can still pursue them if they feel they are possibly going to collect them in the future, but this will be gut-check time for both of you. Your writing some claims off is going to hurt, but they weren't coming in anyway.

Doing this shows your insurance person that you are going to help them move towards hitting this number on a regular basis.

You might consider moving it to 5% of over 90 (which is completely up to you) or you might want to change it over a few months. Spiff your person on 5% for the first 3-6 months knowing that it will be spiffed off of 3% going forward. You'll find your insurance person fighting harder for claims, they will keep a better check on your front desk to make sure they are verifying insurance, and you will collect a higher % of your claims and deposit more money.

Appendix IV – Bonus for Offices with Scheduled Appointments

Spiffing Your Front Desk

The most effective spiff for your front desk is how full they keep your schedule. For this to have its largest impact on your bottom line, you are going to have to monitor it well. Let me explain.

I recommend a spiff based on a % of your schedule being filled. For example, if you are a practice with a healthy patient base, you may be scheduled out for a week or so at the time. That is a great problem to have, and you want to address that problem by seeing as many comprehensive eye exams in one day as you can. So, pick a % that is going to make your staff work hard and efficiently. For sake of demonstration, I'm going to choose 95% as the goal. You can choose whatever you think will make your staff work hard but also be reachable.

To get to 95%, several things need to be in place. First and foremost, there has to be a schedule template. Staff must be instructed as to where and when they place exams, office visits, and follow ups on your schedule. Never leave it to the whims of your front desk person. Though they may mean well, without motivation and accountability, your staff is always going to schedule your staff as to what is convenient for them. Without a template, you will almost never have a full schedule at the end of a day, and I guarantee you that you won't have busy schedules on Friday afternoons.

Your job is to tell the front desk where and when to schedule; their job is to fill that schedule.

There are as many sample templates as there are business in this world, so I offer one merely to get you to examine your day and make the determination for yourself. To begin, ask yourself this question, "How many comprehensive eye exams can I see in one uninterrupted hour?" I've seen one doctor choose anywhere between 1 and 6. For the sake of this discussion, let's go with 3.

Now look at when you start your day, when you go to lunch, and when you want to leave. The first 20 minutes of your day should be follow up and medical exams. The 20 minutes prior to lunch should be the same, the first 20 minutes after lunch, and the final 20 minutes of your day should be the same. With 10 minutes for each appointment, you have 8 slots each day to see follow ups and sick-eyes. That is plenty. The rest of the day should be reserved for comprehensive exams which offer you your greatest opportunity for revenue.

Let's say you open your doors at 8:00am and close at 5:00. You take lunch from 12:00pm to 1:00 pm. Then your template looks like this:

Time	Appointment
8:00 am	Follow Up/Sick Eye
8:10 am	Follow Up/Sick Eye
8:20 am	Comprehensive Exam
8:40 am	Comprehensive Exam
9:00 am	Comprehensive Exam
9:20 am	Comprehensive Exam

9:40 am	Comprehensive Exam
10:00 am	Comprehensive Exam
10:20 am	Comprehensive Exam
10:40 am	Comprehensive Exam
11:00 am	Comprehensive Exam
11:20 am	Comprehensive Exam
11:40 am	Follow Up/Sick Eye
11:50 am	Follow Up/Sick Eye
12:00 pm	Lunch
1:00 pm	Follow Up/Sick Eye
1:10 pm	Follow Up/Sick Eye
1:20 pm	Comprehensive Exam
1:40 pm	Comprehensive Exam
2:00 pm	Comprehensive Exam
2:20 pm	Comprehensive Exam
2:40 pm	Comprehensive Exam
3:00 pm	Comprehensive Exam
3:20 pm	Comprehensive Exam
3:40 pm	Comprehensive Exam
4:00 pm	Comprehensive Exam
4:20 pm	Comprehensive Exam
4:40 pm	Follow Up/Sick Eye
5:00 pm	Follow Up/Sick Eye

With this schedule, you can see 20 comprehensive exams a day and 8 follow ups and sick eyes. Now, that may look like a sweet schedule, but recognize that in a typical 20 business day month, you would see 400 comprehensive exams. That would be sweet if you have the patient base. If you feel that number is one you would have to grow into, then adjust your schedule to 2 full exams and hour (depending upon where you start and start, that would give you 13-15 exams a day and 260-300 exams a month).

Okay, spiffs for your front desk can be made up of a various items, but I like to go food for weekly and money for monthly. If 95% occupancy is your goal on a 3 exams an hour schedule, then the entire office gets lunch if you see 95 exams during the week. If you already have a lunch scheduled for Monday because of optical, great, then the staff gets lunch Monday and Tuesday. A monthly spiff is easy to come up with; just remind yourself of the additional income you are enjoying because of the fuller schedule.

About the Author

Gordon Duncan is an award-winning educator, salesman, teacher, manager, and writer. He has taught in the public school system, lobbied for school's accreditation, managed eye clinics, led sales' teams, and also publishes books on theology, church, and culture.

In addition, he writes regularly on running and spiritual issues through http://www.examiner.com/evangelical-in-raleigh/gordon-duncan,and http://www.examiner.com/running-in-raleigh/gordon-duncan.

You can find out more about his philosophies for the eye industry at www.practiceprogress.com and his thoughts on church and culture at www.jgordonduncan.com.

He has been happily married to Amy for over 15 years and is the proud father of 3 wonderful girls.

He is a graduate of East Carolina University and Reformed Theological Seminary.